Psychological effects of a pandemic

I0505403

# ANTIVIRUS

How to Build Resilience and
Overcome Fear

ROBERT LEDWARD

**Copyright © 2020 Robert J. Ledward**

**All rights reserved**

This book is not intended as a substitute for the medical advice of physicians. The reader should regularly consult a physician in matters relating to his/her health and particularly with respect to any symptoms that may require diagnosis or medical                                              attention.

*"Many times, the thought of fear itself is greater than what it is we fear."*

*(Idowu Koyenikan)*

### What Did You Think of Antivirus?

First of all, thank you for purchasing Antivirus.
If you enjoyed this book and found some benefit in
reading this, I'd like to hear from you and hope that you
could take some time to post a review on Amazon. Your
feedback and support will help this author to greatly
improve his writing craft for future projects and make
this book even better.

Enjoy the reading!

# TABLE OF CONTENTS

# INTRODUCTION

I first heard about the coronavirus when I saw news programs showing pictures of Wuhan in trouble. I watched with concern as the virus spread rapidly, and the infections increased exponentially. I never believed that it would affect me personally, but this invisible enemy soon arrived in Europe, where I was attending a conference.

I experienced the first phenomena of collective psychosis - people cleared grocery store shelves as if they were in a war, with fear in their eyes.

I painstakingly inquired into the disease and understood that there was no need to panic, but the danger shouldn't be underestimated. Knowledge is the best tool against fear.

I believe this virus will spread and reach other countries around the world, including the USA. We must be ready, not only with regards to our health, but also with regards to how it affects us psychologically.

In this guide I will share what I have learned. It is not intended to be a medical treatise or to replace directions and advice from competent authorities. In this guide, you will find a set of suggestions to restore calmness to your life, while being ready to face this new enemy that, perhaps because it is invisible and unknown, makes us afraid.

# EPIDEMICS IN HUMAN HISTORY

Over the span of history, a few sicknesses and scourges have hit the human populace so much that we frequently wonder if the end of mankind will happen sooner than we anticipated. The loss of life and a large portion of these pestilences that have been recorded have assaulted humankind and at times all the while, changed the course of history.

Of all ailments that have undermined civic establishments on earth, cholera, little pox, bubonic plague, little pox, and flu are probably the deadliest executioners throughout the entire existence of humanity. A portion of these scourges has made us wonder if every one of these maladies is flagging the end of whole human advancements.

As the earth keeps on getting progressively populated, there is a steadily expanding rate in the quantity of irresistible infection also, from the Antonine Plague to the current COVID-19 occasion.

A portion of the pandemics and scourges that have hit the human populace from ancient to present day times are talked about underneath:

ANTONINE PLAGUE (165 AD)

This plague was likewise alluded to as the Plague of Galen. It was an old pandemic that influenced the Asian Minor, Egyptians, Greeks, and Italians and it is accepted to have been either little pox or measles. In spite of the fact that the genuine reason is as yet not known, the pandemic was said to have come back to Rome by Roman warriors coming back from Mesopotamia around 165AD. As per history, the loss of life brought about by the Antonine Plague is supposed to be around 5 million individuals just as the obliteration of the whole Roman armed force.

THE BLACK DEATH (1346-1353)

Another horrible pandemic that hit the world was the Bubonic Plague. Somewhere in the range of 1346 and 1353, an episode of the plague attacked the Europeans, Africans, and the Asians. The loss of life is supposed to be around 75 – 200 million individuals. The vast majority accepted that the plague initially spread from Asia however a few theories propose that the plague probably hopped mainlands because of the insects living on the rodents that possessed the dealerships. The slippery bacterium was said to have crushed three continents afterwards.

## THIRD CHOLERA PANDEMIC (1852-1860)

A great many people consider this the deadliest of every one of the seven cholera pandemics to hit human development. The third cholera pandemic kept going from 1852 to 1860 and like other cholera pandemics; this one was likewise accepted to have started from India. It at that point spread from the Ganges River Delta through Asia, Europe, North America, and Africa and caused the demise of in excess of a million people. A British doctor, John Snow had the option to find the methods for transmission of the infection was through debased water while he was on task in a poor region of London.

## HIV/AIDS PANDEMIC (1981 TILL PRESENT)

Since its disclosure, AIDS has killed more than 35 million individuals. HIV, the infection answerable for the malady called AIDS was supposed to have been created from a chimpanzee infection that happened to reach the human populace in West Africa in the 1920s. From that point forward, the infection advanced over the globe and AIDS turned into a pandemic by the late 2oth century. There is no known fix however with the assistance of meds created during the 1990s, individuals who experience the ill effects of the infection can live more and have a typical life expectancy as long as they experience ordinary treatment.

### COVID-19 (2019 TILL PRESENT)

The new Coronavirus has created a global panic. From the epicenter of the outbreak, in the Chinese city of Wuhan, the infection has spread rapidly and many are fearful of contracting the disease.

# AN INVISIBLE ENEMY

The new Coronavirus has created a worldwide panic. Those infected are increasing, and nobody feels safe anymore. Let's look at the origin of this pandemic.

Everything appears to link back to Wuhan, the Chinese megalopolis, capital and largest city of Hubei province. It is here that in the last months of 2019, something happened that was the epicenter of this worldwide spread.

Ground zero is thought to have been one of the many fish markets in the city where, alongside fish and seafood, numerous live animals are normally sold, such as snakes, turtles, salamanders, peacocks, porcupines and other wild animals. The animals are intended to be killed and cooked by customers later. The risk of contamination is high because of the lack of basic sanitary standards.

Scientists first identified the snake, then the bat, then the pangolin as the animals that would transmit the disease – mutated in the meantime - to humans.

Another hypothesis indicated that the outbreak was caused by a breach in the Wuhan level 4 biosafety laboratory (BSL-4).

Whatever the origin, the result is that this new virus, easily transmitted, has rapidly spread in this extremely crowded city, giving rise to a contagion that has grown exponentially.

The virus produces symptoms that are often light and easily mistaken for a seasonal flu. Because of this, the disease has spread through apparently asymptomatic or slightly symptomatic people, multiplying the number of affected people.

We'll look at something called the R0 factor, which describes communicability and incubation times. This factor has allowed an immediate and very rapid spread that has caused Wuhan and its hospital system to collapse.

The situation seems to have been aggravated by a delay in the discovery and reporting of the new virus by the Chinese authorities, making it impossible to contain the initial outbreak. Unfortunately, the symptoms of the new coronavirus led to a high number of people (an estimated 15% of those infected) needing hospitalization, and a number of these needed intensive care and respiratory assistance.

The overwhelming number of simultaneous cases that erupted in Wuhan led to a lack of beds and hospitals, an unsustainable situation despite the construction of two new hospital complexes built in only a few days.

Eventually, the Chinese government implemented the largest quarantine in history.

They imposed restrictions on transportation and the movement of people across the city of Wuhan, a metropolis with a population of 11 million people. The restrictions were then extended to the rest of the province. A region with nearly 60 million inhabitants was locked down under armed surveillance.

The Chinese New Year festivities were extended, and the government recommended that Chinese citizens not leave the country, and work as much as possible from home. All domestic transportation by bus, train and plane was discontinued and unprecedented measures were taken to halt the spread of the disease.

Let's try to understand what this new coronavirus is, to which they have given the name SARS-CoV-2.

What are the characteristics of this invisible enemy that has caused so much fear?

Coronaviruses are a large family of viruses that can cause various infections, from the common cold to more serious diseases such as Middle Eastern respiratory syndrome (MERS) and severe acute respiratory syndrome (SARS).

The disease caused by the new coronavirus is called, "COVID-19" (where "CO" stands for corona, "VI" for virus, "D" for disease and "19" indicates the year in which it occurred).

Coronaviruses are parasitic microorganisms, capable of replicating exclusively within the cells of other organisms. They use RNA as genetic material, present with a single strand.

The name of the virus derives from the classic shape seen under the electron microscope. "Nails" dot the external surface of the virus and give it the appearance of a crown.

Coronaviruses are present in many animal species. On rare occasions, they mutate into a form that allows them to infect humans.

This contagion was accidental, perhaps due to the fact that these people had been close to bats or other infected wild animals and accidentally came into contact with their bodily fluids or excrements.

When we talk about a "new coronavirus", it means that we are faced with a new strain that has never been found in humans.

This implies that none of us have antibodies and are therefore the virus will more easily infect us.

Vaccines are available to protect more susceptible people from influenza, but that is not the case for this new virus. It spreads quickly and easily.

# RESILIENCE: ADAPTIVE ABILITY TO CRITICAL SITUATIONS

Perhaps the hardest unavoidable truth is that we will all experience misfortune, somehow. Resilience causes us to manage affliction – it is a quality that permits the individuals who have been struck somewhere around life's cruelty to return more grounded or if nothing else, as solid as they were previously. Resilient individuals would prefer not to let challenges or their disappointments overload them; they figure out how to rise.

Numerous analysts will concur that a portion of the elements that make an individual resilient incorporates an inspirational mentality, a sound degree of good faith, the capacity to manage and control feelings just as the capacity to abstain from considering the inability to be a misfortune yet as a type of accommodating input and as a solid helper for progress. Analysts who have enjoyed broad research share the supposition that confidence assists obscure with excursion the effect of weight on such an individual's brain and body as they experience a large group of upsetting encounters.

In contrast to the conviction of a great many people, everybody can achieve some degree of resilience – it's anything but a supernatural quality however a propensity that takes genuine subjective work to transcend the hardship of the real world. On later occasions, there are a few confirmations that demonstrate that the components of strength can be created and developed. The facts confirm that sooner or later in our lives we as a whole experience mishap yet it is additionally evident that considerably after setback, strong individuals can push ahead and change course in a positive light to accomplish their objectives.

How Can One Bounce Back After A Challenge Of Misfortune?

The fundamental reason strength expects to accomplish is to ensure we traverse the agony and frustration we regularly experience without giving these everyday hardships the instruments to pound our spirits. Genuinely, nobody could ever disclose to you that skipping back is simple yet inquiry about has kept on revealing the insider facts of resilient individuals and how they can persevere after they endure an injury, for example, losing a friend or family member, losing a vocation, or some other sort of mishap.

Would you be able to state that all your expert and individual mishaps are because of your own deficiency? The appropriate response is a capital "No" however you can choose to recognize and pay special mind to factors that may be adding to your deficiency. These outside or interior factors as the case might be could be explicit and brief. The last quality has been ascribed to individuals who have more prominent degrees of strength.

Accounts of individuals who have experienced excruciating conditions and can defeat them are sufficient proof that fiascos can be survived. The initial step to building up a solid degree of versatility is to comprehend that to fall flat is profoundly human however we ought not to overlook that as people, we were brought into the world with the inborn ability to review, gain from and rise above disappointment.

The lessons we can find from our disappointments have suggestions for quietude, development, and compassion. One doesn't have to profess to his or herself that it's a joy to come up short or that he can disregard the disappointment that these disappointments bring however so as to be versatile, one needs to begin tolerating the sentiments that disappointment brings, become inquisitive about these disappointments and fight the temptation to pass judgment on oneself.

At the point when one starts to ace and practice these basic aptitudes, you are on the solid shower to getting strong. Other than developing better authority over our feelings, rehearsing these aptitudes assist us with seeing lessons that will keep us from committing similar errors all over again.

# THE CORRECT APPROACH TO EMERGENCIES

Envision you are strolling home late in obscurity then you begin to hear delicate, snapping hints of people or somebody sneaking up behind you or you hear the sound of a person or thing stepping on dry leaves close by. The first thing you'll notice is your heart dashing and beating intensely then you would potentially start to wonder who or what prowls inside the shadows. Right now, can you say you are afraid or anxious?

Once in a while, it's difficult to educate the contrast between fear and anxiety. The difference between these feelings is frequently mistaken and even within the literature of psychology; somebody who is familiar with the terms used in psychology will see that the words are utilized reciprocally.

We as individuals fear something, right? The fear of the obscure, feelings of dread of death, fear of blankness and devastation or fear of oblivion, etc. They're totally understood as fear however in truth, they're really experienced as feelings of nervousness and anxiety. The greater part of the individuals is of the feeling that fears are an outcome of tension issues. It's then not a criminal offence to make reference to the fact that fear and anxiety are important to differentiate to the point that it should now be possible to do so.

Fear and anxiety can rise above into actions that make us cautious about some specific circumstances and situations. They regularly fill in as defense mechanisms. Talking by and large terms, Fear is characterized as our response to immediate circumstances that undermine our wellbeing and security. This feeling triggers our feeling of cognizance that we'd prefer to keep ourselves from getting hurt at whatever point we find ourselves in a circumstance such is reality undermining.

It is such that the thought of fight or flight is considered to be a reaction activated by fear. As opposed to fear, anxiety might be an inclination of misery activated by something as a rule not explicit but rather most importantly they're both activated because of perceived risk or threat. The least difficult approach to decide fear, according to research carried out by certain researchers is by deciding if non-evasion is imminent or if in that circumstance, such an individual's activity is seen to be in a state of harmony with shirking or departure.

Generally, the presence of evasion in the conduct of such an individual will indicate fear while rather than fear, a restless individual will be essentially alert yet doesn't demonstrate any indications of shirking. As far as evolution is concerned, we'll understand that for a long time, fear has shielded people from predators and bunches of life-imperiling experiences.

Prudence, on the contrary, is considered an ethicalness that pervades a person's character. As indicated by Aristotle, Prudence is what motivates good and appropriate conduct. In the present day, prudence is pretty much likely identified with foresight – somebody is viewed as prudent when the person in question thinks before they act or all the more properly when somebody ruminates over the aftereffects of their moves before making them.

While some look at prudence as righteousness, others accept that prudence is pretty much kind of an absence of motivation as well as inspiration. Prudence includes a positive side and everything must do with foreknowledge; when you profoundly think about the circumstance to decide the ramifications of your activities. Being prudent and having the intensity of foreknowledge is indispensable for making choices.

Reasonability doesn't mean one is incautious as it is goodness firmly identified with insight, capacity to think about circumstances and poise. There are some of a few confusions of Prudence yet it's not fear. Prudence is actually a duty.

# GLOBAL SPREAD

Despite the containment measures put in place by China and other countries around the world to avoid importing the virus, the spread has been inevitable. Infected people are now present in many countries around the world, giving rise to many outbreaks of contagion.

Let's take a look at why the new coronavirus is so contagious and why it spreads, despite the actions taken by governments around the world.

It is important to analyze what is-called the R0 factor. This is the basic reproduction number, which indicates the degree of contagiousness of a virus. Put simply, it indicates the average number of people that an infected person will in turn infect. If this number is less than 1, the epidemic is doomed to end on its own. If this number is equal to 2, it means that each infected person will infect 2 people, who in turn infect two others, resulting in exponential growth. The R0 factor for the new coronavirus is estimated to be between 2 and 2.5. This is higher than traditional flu and therefore more contagious.

Another factor to consider is the incubation time. This number indicates the period of time that passes between the infection and the appearance of the first symptoms. In the case of COVID-19, the time span is about 14 days, although the symptoms of the infection typically occur around the fifth day.

Starting in late 2019, Coronavirus began to spread outside of China. Beginning in nearby Japan, the virus then spread to South Korea, Italy, Iran, and Singapore. New cases were quickly seen in Africa, Russia and the United States. Medical staff on a cruise ship, the Diamond Princess, also diagnosed positive cases on board, and the ship was kept moored in quarantine while the infections continued to multiply despite the isolation measures imposed on the ship's passengers.

The World Health Organization has been following the evolution of the pandemic, gradually raising the alarm level and spreading guidelines people should follow.

How is this coronavirus transmitted from person to person? The primary cause of contagion is close contact with an infected person, through the droplets of saliva that are transmitted by coughing or sneezing. For this reason, contact with people who show flu symptoms should be avoided. Try to stay three feet away from people who are at risk, because the virus seems to also be transmitted, though less easily, by a person who has contracted it but appears asymptomatic.

It also appears that the virus can survive for several hours on surfaces, so it is even possible to become infected by touching contaminated surfaces, then touching your hands, mouth or nose before washing them thoroughly.

Most virologists and epidemiologists are convinced that the new coronavirus will spread worldwide. Our ability to contain it will depend on targeted isolation actions, and the implementation of hygiene rules will determine its slowdown. As for its virulence, it is hoped that over time this will decrease and, like the common flu, it will slow down and possibly disappear completely during the warmer months.

Let's examine the symptoms of this disease, see how it is diagnosed, and discover what the current treatment is.

First of all, let us clarify that even though someone may call it a simple flu, it is not. It's relevant to notice that numbers of cases observed in China and other countries indicate that the majority of people now infected are affected by a mild form that can actually be superimposed on the common cold or seasonal flu. Another part need hospitalization, and about ten percent need assistance in intensive care units. Mortality is around 2%, though the data is still being evaluated.

Therefore, we can say that we are not facing a severe epidemic and that mortality, although higher than the flu, is not particularly worrying. The disease appears to be lethal mainly for the elderly or those debilitated by other serious diseases, such as diabetes, heart disease or cancer. It also seems clear that, fortunately, children are spared and if infected, show very mild symptoms.

The main problem we see is related to the speed of the spread and the ability of the health systems of various nations to withstand the impact. The real risk is that the number of available beds in intensive care units will not be sufficient for the number of people who need them. This has become a reality in China and in several other countries.

Like other respiratory diseases, the main symptoms of Covid-19, can be mild. Patients can have minor symptoms such as colds, sore throats, dry coughs, conjunctivitis and fevers, or more severe symptoms such as pneumonia and breathing difficulties. In some cases, as mentioned, people develop no symptoms or malaise.

Diagnosis is made through an oropharyngeal swab, with the analysis carried out in the laboratory. Because this a new virus affecting humans, there are currently no vaccines being studied. Any new vaccines will need several months to be made available. Antibiotics are not effective since they only act on bacterial infections and not on viruses.

Treatment is therefore currently based on patient symptoms. Our bodies must be the ones to create the antibodies that will fight the virus. However, some positive results have been obtained through the use of antiviral drugs designed for the HIV and Ebola viruses. Specific therapies are currently being studied.

Patients who have recovered show complete freedom from symptoms and a swab test will be negative. Blood tests can verify the presence of antibodies, though the first recurrences of the disease have been found in China.

Although Covid-19 is not an extremely lethal virus, it should not be underestimated. It should not be mistaken for a common flu, despite the fact that the symptoms are similar for the majority of those infected. Because this is a new virus, and a vaccine is not currently available, it is difficult if not impossible to protect the most susceptible populations ahead of time, since these groups will suffer the most severe effects of this new pandemic.

# PSYCHOLOGICAL REACTION
# OF DENIAL

Denial is considered to be one among many coping mechanisms and intrinsically, it gives one time to adjust to situations that prove to be harmful or life-threatening. What many of us don't know is that when one is in denial for too long, it can affect treatment or one's ability to tackle tough situations.

Indeed, everybody is usually trying to guard themselves but once you begin to guard yourself by refusing to acknowledge the presence of a threat in your life, you're in denial and in such situation, you're just aiming to ignore the very fact and also the hard truth that something awfully bad is going on in your life. Most of the time, short-term denial may be a positive reaction to some situations as you'll have enough time to adjust and familiarize yourself with a painful or stressful situation but once you push things too far, denial its3elf features a dark side with really ugly consequences.

Everyone understands that it's very normal to feel like refusing to believe that something is wrong somewhere – one of the various ways to deal with emotional conflicts, stress, anxiety, threatening information and situations and what have you. We are often in denial about things that make us feel powerless and vulnerable like financial problems, career problems, unemployment, addictions, eating disorders, personality disorders or maybe relationship conflicts and once you are in denial, you've got the tendency to either downplay the possible side effects of such issues or perhaps, avoid facing the facts of the matter.

But there are times where being in denial is useful and there are situations where it isn't – a brief period of denial allows our inner consciousness to soak up disheartening and discomforting information at a pace that won't cause you to fall under a psychological tailspin. this sort of denial is especially helpful in responding to shocking situations. during this situation, your mind has absorbed the likelihood of an imminent threat but as your mind accepts this possibility, you begin to seek out a solution carefully and rationally and then take eventually take action by seeking help.

But what if you never leave to seek help? What if you're in denial for so long, it prevents you from doing the proper thing or taking cautionary measures? At this stage, being in denial is bad for you or anyone. it's important to understand that denial should only be a short-lived measure. When faced with an overwhelming situation, it's okay to want to take some time to work through your situation and adapt to new circumstances but being in denial doesn't change things or assist you out of it.

If you're not strong enough to make progress in handling a stressful situation on your own, then you're probably stuck within the denial phase and therefore the smartest thing to do is to seek a mental health provider. Such persons will assist you in finding healthy ways to deal with your situation instead of pretending to be okay or that what you're going through doesn't exist in the least.

# FREEDOM OF PERSON AND COLLECTIVE WELL-BEING

Pandemics are alluded to as huge scope flare-ups of irresistible infections that achieve a dynamic ascent in the pace of mortality and grimness over a wide geographic zone and trigger host of huge financial, social and political interruptions. In basic terms, a pandemic is a circumstance whereby an irresistible ailment compromises a nation or the entire world.

Some proof has proposed that there is an expansion in the pace of pandemics in the course of the only remaining century because of worldwide travel and incorporation, urbanization and changes in land use just as investigation of the regular habitat. The reality remains that these patterns will increase and all things considered noteworthy strategy consideration has focused on the need to angle out and limit potential flare-ups that could cause pandemics including growing and continuing speculations that will fill in as hardware to fabricate and create readiness and wellbeing limit.

The universal network is continually gaining ground in planning for and relieving the effects of pandemics. Regardless of these enhancements and arrangements, it is as yet a reality that there are as yet recognizable holes and difficulties in the worldwide pandemic readiness. Numerous pandemic flare-ups, particularly the West Africa Ebola Epidemic in 2014, have uncovered these shortcomings including holes identified with the auspicious event of the sickness, accessibility of fundamental consideration, isolate, seclusion and readiness outside the wellbeing area.

The universal network has arranged a rundown of suggested activities for previously, during and after a pandemic. Thusly, they can handle the spread of the pandemic successfully and all things considered, such measures limit the singular opportunity for the aggregate prosperity of the overall population. It is known to everybody that diminishing the spread of an ailment will depend entirely and fundamentally on expanding the social separation between individuals just as restricting contact between people.

There are diverse preventative estimates that are essential to the aggregate prosperity and wellbeing of the entire world. Such measures are singular/family, cultural, and universal travel. Antiviral, immunizations and different pharmaceuticals demonstrate helpful in lessening the spread of such pandemics. A portion of the Individual/family unit estimates will incorporate hazard correspondence, singular cleanliness, individual insurance and home consideration of contaminated casualty just as an isolate of contacts.

A portion of the cultural level measures include an adjustment in the conduct of the populace, for example, curfews and development bans, numerous area associations may be orchestrated just as an assembly of assets, limitation of development, solid correspondence and media support. Global travel estimates will be planned for postponing the section of pandemic illnesses into nations that have not been influenced. It will likewise affect universal traffic and exchange as nations should adjust decreasing the dangers to the open heath while maintaining a strategic distance from obstruction with worldwide exchange and traffic.

The utilization of pharmaceuticals will likewise help guarantee the anticipation and treatment of pandemic flare-ups. It is essential to include that effective anticipation or potential treatment of auxiliary or previous conditions will be fundamental in decreasing the spread of disease.

# HOW CAN WE PROTECT OURSELVES?

Globalization has made it impossible to stem the virus. Movements for work, tourism, and trade have led to the emergence of outbreaks in many countries of the world. When an infection is discovered in a new geographical area, every effort is made to identify the so-called "index patient," or "zero patient." It is important to be able to immediately map the people who came into contact with him or her, and isolate them so that they do not transmit the infection to others. When identification of the index patient is impossible, the focus of health care authorities turns to curbing the outbreak by isolating the entire affected area and preventing people from leaving. For example, this is what happened in Italy, where an entire area of the Lombardy region was isolated and quarantined.

For individuals, this basic protective action is linked to prevention. It is extremely important to diligently follow the rules set up by the World Health Organization and by the health authorities of your own country.

Great importance is given to personal hygiene and the recommendation to avoid contact between people. We can summarize some tips in the following 10 rules:

1. Wash your hands often.

2. Avoid close contact with people suffering from acute respiratory infections.

3. Do not touch your eyes, nose and mouth with your hands.

4. Cover your mouth and nose if you sneeze or cough.

5. Do not take antiviral drugs or antibiotics, unless they are prescribed by your doctor.

6. Clean surfaces with chlorine-based or alcohol-based disinfectants.

7. Use a mask if you suspect you are sick or if you are assisting sick people.

8. Remember that products made in China and parcels received from China are not dangerous.

9. Pets do not spread the new coronavirus.

10. If you have any questions, contact the national health system according to the guidelines they provide.

These rules are logical, understandable and universal. If everyone remains committed to them, even if it requires small changes in our habits, it will be possible to put a brake on the spread of the virus. It will allow us the time necessary to expand the capacity of countries to control it.

Protective masks deserve a separate discussion. Many people are using them. In the most affected areas, they were hoarded, and they have become nearly unavailable in many areas. Let's discuss their usefulness, and the different kinds of masks available.

Professional protection masks that are actually capable of protecting against viruses are used by healthcare professionals. However, it is necessary to know the correct way to use them. Used incorrectly, they can be counterproductive.

Many people continue to buy disposable surgical masks, and several pharmacies report having run out of these products. Be careful, though. These masks are capable of protecting against biological sprays or secretions, but not from fine aerosols, such as those of viruses. Therefore, these masks are more useful for preventing the spread of viruses from patients who are already sick, rather than for protecting healthy people.

There are different types of masks on the market, depending on the function they perform:

- The simple masks used for hygiene purposes by workers in the food industry are not designed to protect the wearer's respiratory tract. They cannot offer a guarantee of protection from infection.

- Surgical masks are designed to reduce the risk of infection among healthcare professionals. There are different types, with an increasing degree of protection depending on the number of filter layers. They are useful because they protect against heavier splashes and secretions, but they are not guaranteed to protect against the finer vapors from an infected person.

- Masks equipped with filters are the only devices capable of giving some protection from viruses. The filtering efficiency of each different mask is indicated with the abbreviation FF, from P1 to P3. The FFP2 and P3 masks, which have a filtering efficiency of 92% and 98% respectively, are the most suitable for protection from viruses, provided that, as we said, you know how to use them.

One piece of advice we would like to give you is to get a hand-sanitizing gel, useful for always keeping your hands disinfected. Even this product has become almost impossible to find in the areas affected by the epidemic.

# PSYCHOLOGICAL CONSEQUENCES OF ISOLATION AND QUARANTINE

In our current reality where COVID-19 and numerous other savage pandemics have shaken the earth, it a preventative measure to ask that individuals remain limited to forestall the spread of such irresistible maladies however actually very few individuals would seize the chance of being kept.

In November 2018, Rich Alati, an expert poker player in the US wager $100,000 that he could make due for 30 days, alone and in the all-out dimness. He was then kept to a little, totally dim room, confined with only a bed, ice chest, and restroom however he was unable to keep going the month all alone. Following 20 days, Alati arranged his discharge and took a payout of US$62,400. We may imagine that we can get by in segregation yet we are unconscious of the various negative impacts related to social detachment and extraordinary disengagement.

Rich Alati's aftermath from his wager is verification that social confinement can effectively affect our psyche and bodies. Alati announced that he encountered a significant huge measure of various symptoms remembering a change for his rest cycle and regular visualizations. The inquiry at the forefront of your thoughts presently ought to be Why Is Isolation So Difficult For Us to Withstand?

As people, we are for the most part social animals. Numerous individuals who have at one point or the other, lived in seclusion, for example, specialists and pilgrims have announced that being forlorn is the hardest an aspect of their responsibilities. Yossi Ghinsberg, an Israeli who endure weeks alone in the Amazon affirmed that depression was what he endured the most and that he even made nonexistent companions stay with himself.

It is regularly horrible to live in disengagement since dejection accomplishes more harm than great to both our psychological well-being and physical wellbeing. Individuals who are socially detached think that its hard to deal with distressful circumstances. They frequently feel discouraged and may have issues with absorbing and handling data. They experience issues in settling on choices just as memory stockpiling and review issues.

Forlorn individuals are increasingly inclined to experience the ill effects of the disease as their body's safe framework reacts to battling infections in an unexpected way. The effects of disconnection are even declined when individuals are being put in truly isolating repressions or conditions, for example, alarm assaults, nervousness, and distrustfulness etc.

The facts confirm that the effects of absolute confinement can be serious, the impacts can be turned around. Reconnecting with different people decreases forlornness and returns us to great mental and physical wellbeing yet frequently than not, individuals who have been held in social confinement without wanting to are inclined to grow long haul medical problems, for example, Post-Traumatic Stress Disorder (PTSD). Asides the pessimistic impacts of segregation, a few people who have remained alone for an all-encompassing timeframe could be said to have encountered self-awareness.

As indicated by Alati, he announced that his experience caused him to acknowledge individuals and life more. It additionally gave him better concentration and consideration and a general sentiment of joy.

# RISKS OF DISCRIMINATION
# AND SOCIAL EXCLUSION

Since the flare-up of the COVID-19 pandemic, the rate at which individuals have been tainted has been said to be continually disturbing to a lot bigger scope every single day. As ahead of schedule as of March 2020, there have been near 90,000 affirmed instances of contaminated individuals in more than 60 nations and among these 90,000, the number of inhabitants in tainted individuals in china alone is supposed to be around 80,000 particularly because this infection previously loosened up in china.

Governments have chosen to take both preparatory and preventative measures in the episode of the infection particularly in nations where the quantities of tainted individuals are perilously high. That being stated, we raise the issue of discrimination. For the sake of aggregate prosperity, individuals have been encouraged to remain inside and isolate yet the COVID-19 apprehensions are being utilized to fuel Sinophobia and hostility to Asian prejudice everywhere including xenophobia. The ramifications of these activities are exceptionally grave particularly on account of the chance of prejudice. There have been accounted for instances of people and enormous gatherings poking bigot fun at Chinese individuals and the crown infection in North America, Europe and especially Asia.

It is even supposed that Asians are forcefully set in isolation exclusively on the premise that they are Asians. There have been reports of bigot features against Asians and situations where individuals are pointlessly being forceful to Asian people particularly the Chinese. In different nations, there have been instances of announced sinophobic/racist aggression to Asian folks and the overwhelming impacts of these activities will additionally make the pandemic spread as individuals who have been tainted won't wind up shouting out or looking for help because of dread of being disparaged and shunned.

The expectation of separation manufactures its own constant pressure. It is extremely upsetting to be an individual from a class that is continually victimized. Stress and despondency are basic reactions of separation and keeping in mind that casualties as of now have enough to bite from the superfluous provocations, they are gradually being fell into another medical issue with likewise grave symptoms. Casualties of separation regularly feel pushed and discouraged and the ramifications of this are suicide or possible death if not dealt with appropriately.

Numerous individuals will concur that segregation is a general medical problem. Irresistible sicknesses are frequently disparaged and this criticism declines endeavours to keep the illness from spreading also entangles determination the board and treatment as casualties or contaminated individuals will think that its difficult to look for help or appropriate clinical consideration.

A few people have even defended their activities as something ordinary and expected during a plague flare-up. A few people have decided to respect their bigotry and bias to be reasonable however in any event when a pandemic episode is a dread promoting, it doesn't legitimize activities of prejudice or xenophobia. Governments and establishments have a significant task to carry out in guaranteeing that whatever approach they may choose, their strategies and orders shouldn't play on bigot generalizations and implications.

Individuals develop inclination about a lot of things without having inside and out information about them. Besides, they don't look for information about these things they have built up a few predispositions against. Along these lines, such predisposition continues developing and spreading like a plague. Everybody has to help right confusions and general wellbeing instruction ought to be made accessible to everybody. More often than not, separation is conceived from dread and misjudging. It is the more typical motivation behind why we oppress a few classes of individuals.

Belittling in a setting like this is out and out off-base and risky not because it triggers bigotry or xenophobia but since it puts everybody in danger.

# OVERCOME ANXIETY AND FEAR

Fear is a normal emotion that can provide benefits to people. It allows you to recognize danger and to respond appropriately. Therefore, don't be ashamed if you are afraid of the coronavirus. It is a real threat that should not be underestimated.

A reasonable amount of fear allows us to activate behaviors necessary for our protection, without panicking.

The coronavirus must not stop us from living, but simply encourage us to adopt the new behaviors that are indicated by world and national health authorities which will allow us to contain this event.

Fear, however, must not become anxiety. It doesn't have to be disproportionate. It must not restrict our lives or compromise our peace-of-mind. Panic makes us less ready to react and more prone to making mistakes.

Why are we so afraid of the new coronavirus? Human beings have always been afraid of what can hurt us, especially when it is unknown or invisible. We listen to the news circulating on the Internet and on social media, and we are led to believe it, even if it is not totally correct or is even completely wrong. The human brain is then predisposed to collective contagion, where we are able to absorb negative emotions, stress, anxiety and panic through our relationship and empathy with others. The fears that emerge can be related to the distant past (plague) or to a more recent event (smallpox), and they are never forgotten.

The best antidote is to remain calm and be rational. Without letting ourselves be influenced by others, especially by those who tend to negatively exaggerate the news, it is necessary to make scientific inquiries, using qualified sources, and to realistically view the extent of the problem. Science and reason are the best helps available against anxiety - often anxiety about the unknown.

It is also important that we continue to dedicate ourselves to the things that make us feel better: reading a book, cooking for the family, watching a movie, listening to music, or dedicating yourself to your hobby. When we are comfortable, our body produces hormones that increase our well-being and counteract any stress hormones.

Avoid excessive information. Spending the day in front of the television news following all the available news programs does not help to calm us down, adds nothing to our understanding, and only increases our level of anxiety.

We recommend using any available time to take a relaxing walk outside. Walking in nature causes us to produce endorphins that help fight stress.

If you already find yourself in a state of anxiety or panic, or even if you believe you need help, it may be advisable to talk to a psychotherapist who can counsel and direct you to an appropriate solution.

We'll conclude with some additional tips that can help us reduce our feelings of anxiety and return our fear to a reasonable and appropriate level. For example, try to eliminate stimulating foods such as alcohol and coffee from your diet - caffeine is also in many common drinks – and choosing fresh foods such as fruits and vegetables instead. Spend time doing physical activity, because it will not help to stay secluded at home. Plan to go walking or cycling, while limiting contact with others at the distances indicated. Start devoting time, perhaps in the evenings, to meditation, which is associated with breathing and relaxation techniques. Learn about the world of plants and herbs, which can offer us invaluable help. An herbal tea with hawthorn, linden, and passionflower can make us feel calmer and more relaxed.

# ECONOMIC CRISE AND THE PSYCHOLOGICAL IMPACT

In 2008, over 750,000 positions were lost each month – a sum of $8.7 million through the span of the downturn. The budgetary vulnerability spreading from the downturn in the land represented a monetary coronary episode as huge money related stun just as the misfortunes to family units from a downturn in the land made financial movement aftermath. In that year, many major modern organizations were inclined to languish chapter 11 and over the worldwide economy, it caused the greatest constriction in outside exchange that the world had ever observed.

A recuperation started in 2009 after an enormous intercession of both money related and monetary approach became possibly the most important factor. That year, work topped at 10 per cent in October. Presently, in 2020, the world is managing the flare-up of COVID-19 also called the crown infection. At this stage, it is too soon to foresee the course of the monetary downturn because of this pandemic yet a financial downturn is unavoidable – it is the main thing that can be unquestionably anticipated.

Because of the isolation and separation strategies everywhere throughout the world, the world's significant businesses are closing down meanwhile which implies processing plants will be shut down, schools will be closed, just as rec centres, bars, schools, universities and cafés will as well. Markers recommend that the US could endure about 1million employment misfortunes every month among now and June. In the oil business, the chance of market withdrawal has made a value war among OPEC, Russia and other shale makers which will pressure the effectively obligated vitality area.

After the pandemic leaves, there will be a requirement for governments to put resources into the general wellbeing foundation. Each nation should get ready to finance and give massively improved reconnaissance just as crisis offices and a significant save limit. All these would serve helpful in creating open doors for profitable spending and making top-notch occupations however as the world is currently confronted with a worldwide wellbeing crisis and the regular enthusiasm for keeping up monetary strength and we as a whole realize that a financial emergency will undoubtedly cause a falling in GDP, evaporating of liquidity and rising/falling in costs because of inflation or deflation.

There are a few occasions of financial emergencies yet we will look at the mental effects of such a downturn or misery, whichever structure the emergencies may take. The monetary emergency is required to trigger optional psychological wellness issues which consequently may cause an expansion in suicide and liquor passing rates.

Nonetheless, the mental impacts of financial emergencies can be deflected by social government assistance and other arrangement measures. For example, dynamic work advertises programs that assist individuals withholding or recapturing their occupations, help fight the emotional wellness impacts of a financial emergency just as family bolster programs. Obligation alleviation projects will help also just as responsive essential consideration administrations. The individual and cultural expenses can be grave if because of financial dangers, joblessness sets in.

# OVERCOMING COLLECTIVE PSYCHOSIS

As we have said, fear is contagious. In these epidemic cases, the real collective psychosis that can occur is very difficult to escape.

According to some studies, the spread of news related to epidemics can touch particularly sensitive triggers in our consciousness. The alarmism of the media, the news offered on every newscast, the perception that the authorities have not fully controlled the situation, and the conflicting opinions exposed by alleged scientists fuel collective fear.

The key role in this psychosis is played by the amygdala, the part of our brain that is involved in the activation of fear and in the perception of new situations. New things are naturally more frightening. For this reason, a virus called influenza, which also causes many deaths every year, makes us less afraid than a new virus we have never heard of before.

Fear stimulates our hypochondria and pushes us towards a dangerous avoidance of the new situation. We tend to lock ourselves in the house, escaping and observing the world only through television and the Internet. Ten deaths announced on one news station become twenty when we listen to the same news on another station. Everything is amplified and magnified, and anxiety becomes contagious.

We are also witnessing an often irrational collective phenomena: the assault on supermarkets to buy basic necessities. Canned goods, staple items, and water disappear from supermarket shelves. Protective masks and disinfectant gels become impossible to find or are available only at astronomical prices.

Official communication from authorities must be carefully managed, not only to avoid omitting critical information, but to avoid fueling this mass psychosis. If it becomes necessary to close schools, theaters, and other public venues, isolate cities, or suspend public events, it can cause anxiety and fear over something perceived as uncontrollable.

Collective phobia can also be transformed into anger, into a hunt for the index patient, and into forms of violence towards infected people. People who are ill with the disease may be seen as responsible for the spread of the epidemic, rather than as victims. People need a real enemy to fight because the invisible enemy causes too much fear. People look at each other with suspicion, those who sneeze are viewed with suspicion, and those who live near affected areas are marginalized.

How can we fight this phenomenon of collective phobia? First of all, authorities must carefully monitor the amount of communication. The media must put aside sensationalism and the desire to broadcast the most alarming news to increase social shares and clicks. Collective responsibility must prevail.

What about us? How can we remain immune from this psychosis? It's not easy, but in this situation we need to use common sense. We have to consider the actual data, explained to us by competent people, without allowing ourselves to be flooded with news that can increase our stress level. We need to maintain an appropriate level of fear and continue to trust in the authorities, especially in the worldwide scientific community. It is essential to follow the directions we are given, without discussion or panic.

Logic helps us understand that crowd behavior is irrational and we must not allow it to affect us. We need to continue living, just with a few more precautions. In 2020, science is stronger than any virus. There is no doubt that this pandemic will be defeated, and that the scientific world will continue to gain strength.

Another prevalent crowd mentality is denial. Reality can be twisted to suggest that the virus is merely a simple flu, and that the public is being manipulated into panic. These strange ideas of secret plots persist, and there will always be people who underestimate the risks by denying them. Some people will question the limitations imposed by the authorities and say that we must start living normally again. These attitudes are wrong as well as dangerous. We have to find the balance between remaining calm and having the correct preventive mindset. The job of the authorities is to dictate the guidelines, and our job is to comply without blowing things out of proportion in any way.

# FIGHTING FAKE NEWS

In times of difficulty, people have to deal with fake news. Fake news is false, invented, misleading or distorted news. The fake news trend has grown with the proliferation of social media and the fact that anyone can publish content on the Internet while pretending to be an expert. The weakest and most naive people will believe what they see and read, which often contributes to further viral propagation of this content through social sharing.

The crisis linked to the coronavirus epidemic is no exception. You'll find all the typical ingredients of an epidemic: accusations, plots, exploitation, and hidden motivations. Not a day goes by that false news hoping to intrigue or generate unjustified alarm is not spread on the Internet. Some examples of false news are that dogs and cats can be healthy carriers of this virus, or that packages and letters from China can bring contagion. There are countless podcasts that report faulty information supported by alleged virologists or respected pediatricians. There are also scams propagated by those who offer to come to the homes of the elderly with the excuse of giving a diagnostic throat swab, but in reality intend to steal some small change.

Fake-news spreads rapidly because it feeds on people's uncertainties and fears, and it creates unjustified alarm. The endless clicking of links that generates advertising profits focuses on the weaknesses of the community and on the fragility of emotions.

How can we defend ourselves? Again, with calm and reason. First of all, by trusting only the authoritative sources and following some simple precautions:

- Don't trust headlines. They are often sensationalized and written in capital letters to attract your attention.

- Double-check the site address (url). Sometimes a fake website can look similar to an authentic one.

- Do research on the source, checking its reliability and its reputation.

- Carefully check photos because they are often counterfeit.

- See if other sources report the same news.

- Make sure that it is not a simple joke, told perhaps in bad taste.

We must try to develop a rational critical sense and avoid sharing news without verifying its validity. By doing this, we will avoid unnecessary alarmism by not being unwitting promoters of misinformation.

# THE CHALLENGE OF SMART
# WORKING AND E-LEARNING

What is smart working? It is another model of work that uses new advancements and improvement of previously existing technology to improve both execution and fulfilment that is acquired from the activity. Individuals regularly mistake the term for collaborating. They are two distinct ideas and the last mentioned; collaborating alludes to sharing workspace and is a term as a rule related to independently employed experts.

The 2 essential thoughts behind the idea of smart working are a progressively gainful method for carrying out the responsibility and the utilization of innovation to complete the activity. The importance of shrewd working methods precisely what it resembles – while generally, separation work is being done in an office space or building, keen working keeps an eye on the activity should be possible anyplace even in a recreation centre, coffeehouse or a carport.

Boris Johnson has informed the public that they should begin telecommuting where conceivable in an offer to contain instances of the continuous UK crown infection since the flare-up of the COVID-19 pandemic. Enormous organizations like Google, JP

Morgan, and Twitter have just started to get ready alternate courses of action to their staff that incorporates mandatory telecommuting. These moves are made as prudent steps with the conviction that keeping workers further separated from one another will support social distancing which will consequently, diminish odds of gathering spread.

As per a review by stage Work human, 33% of the residents of the US are present as of now working remotely. Joe Hirsh, an interchanges master revealed to CNBC that he accepted that the ongoing COVID-19 pandemic flare-up will make telecommuting a potential normal practice. Likewise, as per a worldwide survey by Kantar, information, and bits of knowledge organization, out of 33,000 individuals, 32% of them esteemed a vocation where they could work remotely. A few people share the assessment that telecommuting could be extremely viable for completing some particular undertakings, for example, those that require profound concentration or security because of its touchy nature.

Qun Li, a partner teacher of big business culture at Beijing Jiao Tong University guarantees that since numerous individuals have taken a stab at telecommuting and have found that to be an approach to adjust life and work, there will be more interest however whether representatives will get what they need is exclusively reliant on the kind of work and how group situated it is, he includes.

Businesses that are more in accordance with media and innovation will permit increasingly adaptable timetables and a higher possibility of allowing staff consent to telecommute yet enterprises that require human exertion – that need labourers on location and have a popularity for group coordination will be against working remotely.

Asides the test of smart working, the crown infection is driving a huge number of children into e-learning. As COVID-19 compromises the security of people when united, schools urge understudies to take an interest in social separating through e-learning in meetings from their homes.

One of the conspicuous advantages of concentrating from home is that review can get customized and time can be utilized all the more wisely. The normal conviction is that e-learning can adequately expand the productivity of self-situated considering.

# LET'S TRUST SCIENCE AND STAY CALM

The world economy will be hit hard by the coronavirus. Stock exchanges will suffer and lose billions of dollars, productive enterprises will be weakened, and entire economic sectors, such as tourism, will be crippled to the limits of their ability to withstand. Then the hard work of reconstruction will begin, as things return to normal and confidence reappears. But the world economy will rebound. It will be the first thing people think about once the health emergency ends.

In conclusion, what should we do so we don't give in to fear and pessimism?

As we have seen, we must have the beacon of knowledge as a guide for our steps. We must remain calm and have full confidence in science.

In 2020, science has evolved to the point where we should not fear a virus.

Scientists from around the world are cooperating to find cures and vaccines. Universities, pharmaceutical companies, and researchers work tirelessly with one goal, and the scientific community collaborates with the utmost transparency.

Advanced instruments, computers and artificial intelligence are being used to shorten the waiting period, and I think we can rest assured and be totally confident that a vaccine will be developed soon.

Quality medical care is now available in much of the world. The ability to provide assistance and care has reached standards unimaginable only a few years ago.

But a lot also depends on us. Our commitment can defeat the mathematical models of the spread of contagion. How? First of all, by informing ourselves correctly and choosing authoritative sources. Second, by following the guidelines put into place by political and health authorities, developed so that the infection can slow down its run. Third, by respecting and enforcing personal hygiene rules and avoiding close contact with other people. Fourth, by treating our immune system, the only real defense currently available, through a balanced diet based on fruit and vegetables, rich in vitamins and antioxidants. And last, by reducing personal anxiety and achieving a peaceful and optimistic understanding and vision based on real data.

Fortunately, we are facing an epidemic that is not particularly lethal. The mortality rate is very low and mainly affects elderly and debilitated people. We need to direct our commitment and compassion towards these people. We need to help the weakest people and protect them while the virus spreads, so that they are shielded from a disease that could be dangerous for them. We should also follow the indications that the scientific community and the authorities have given us in order to delay, if not extinguish, the spread of the infection. We owe this to our parents and grandparents.

The first step is to restore our collective health. The economy is the next thing to immediately consider. This pandemic will be remembered in history. But humanity will continue, even stronger than before.